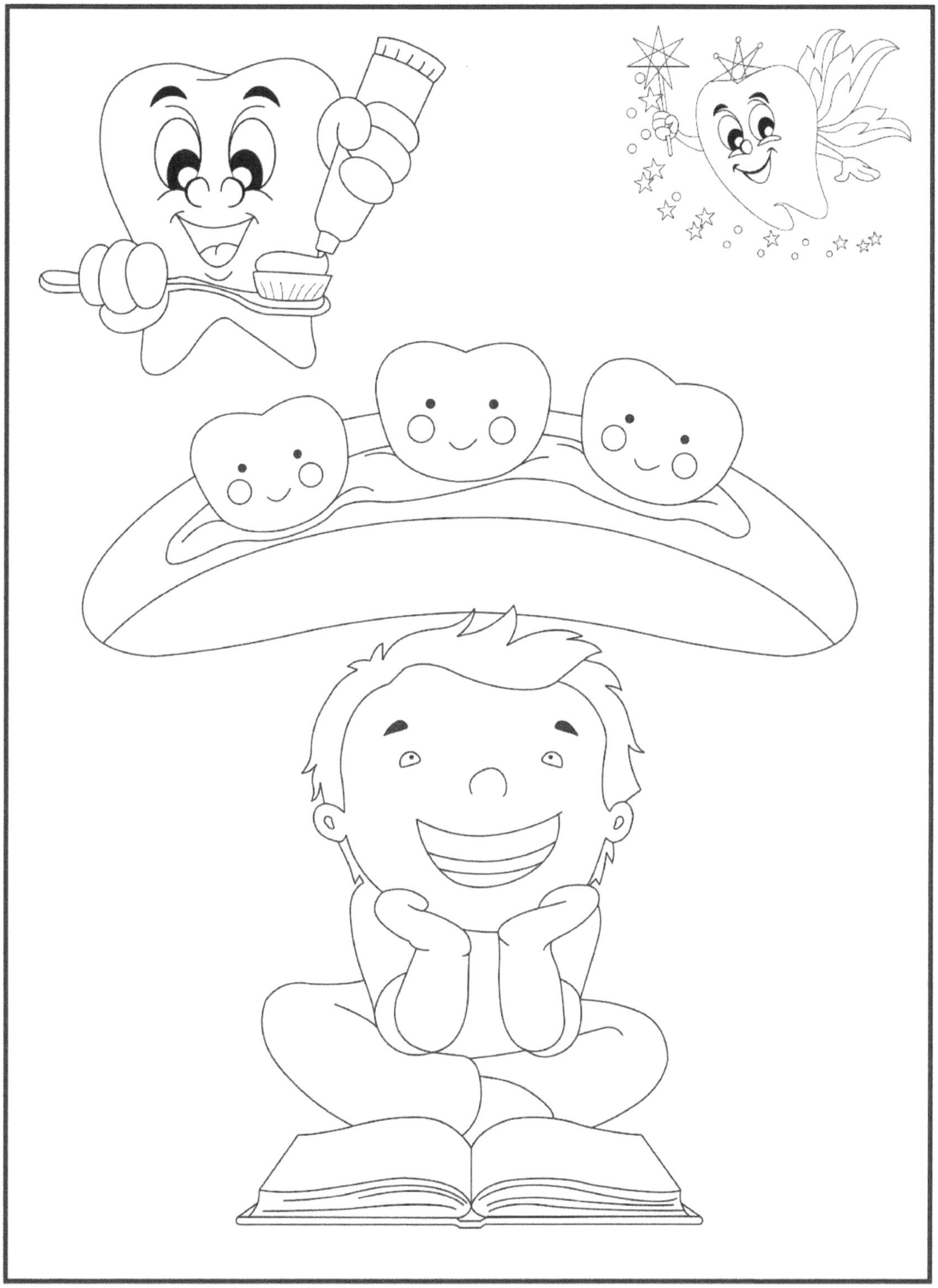

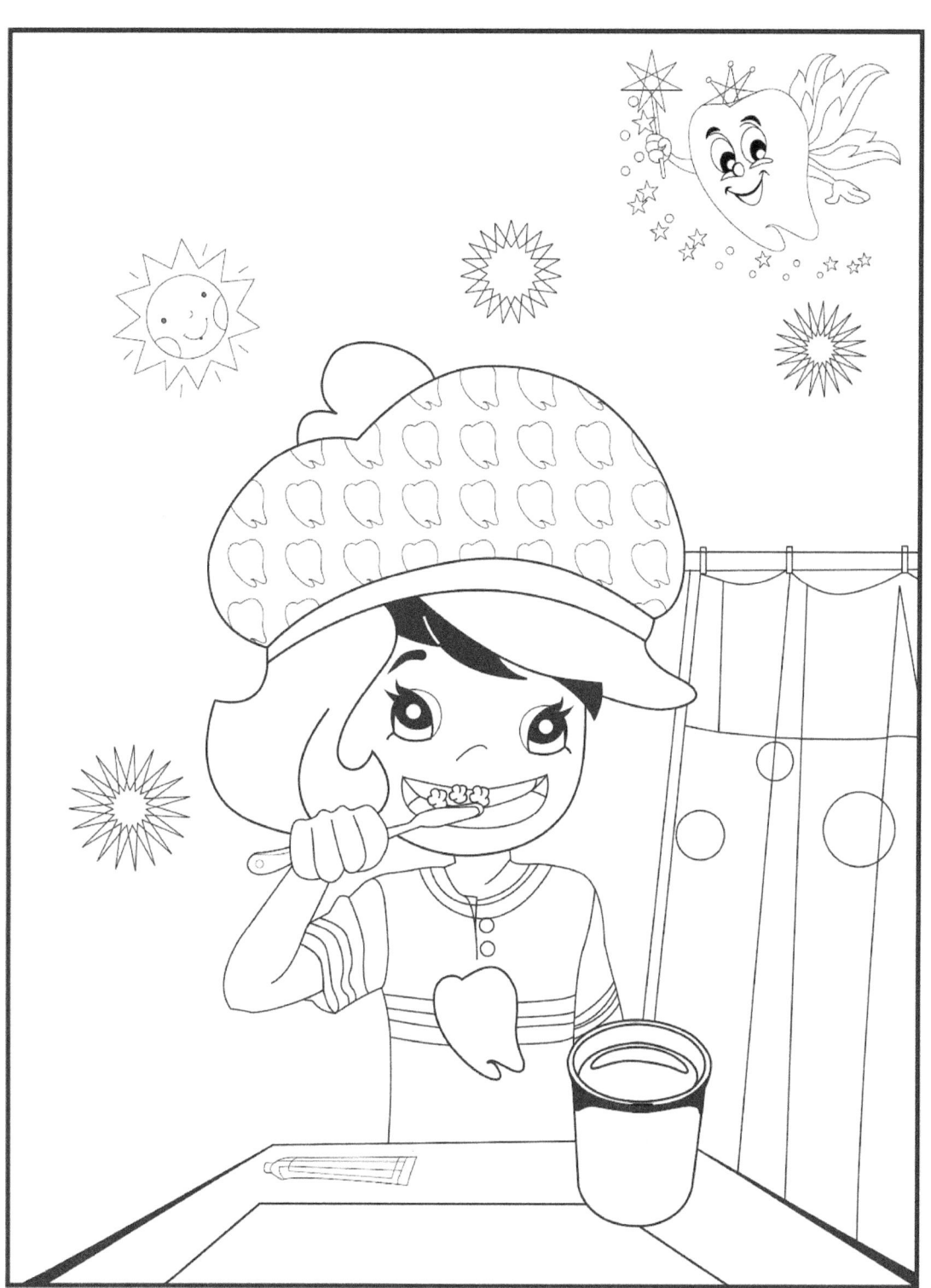

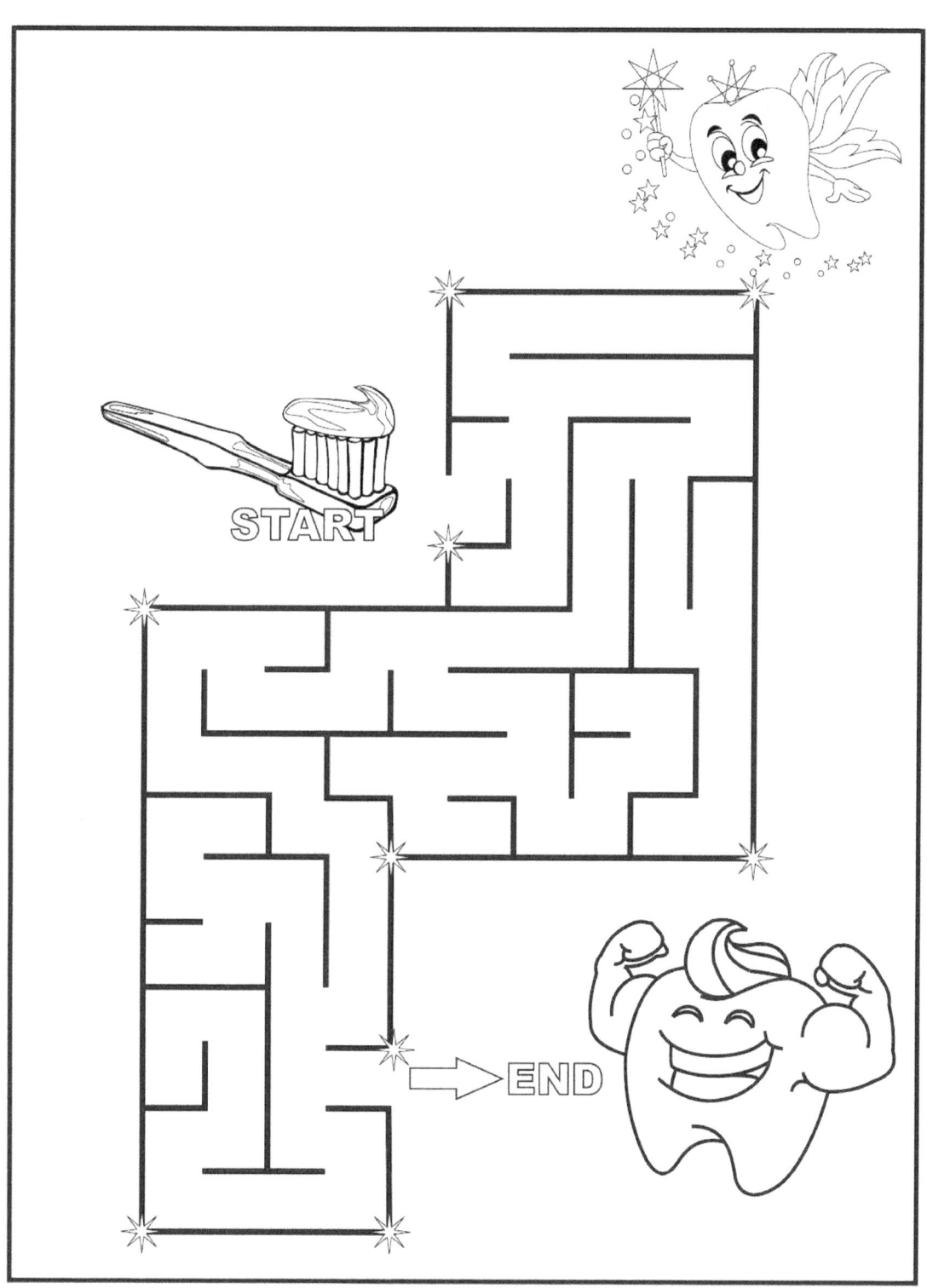

START

END

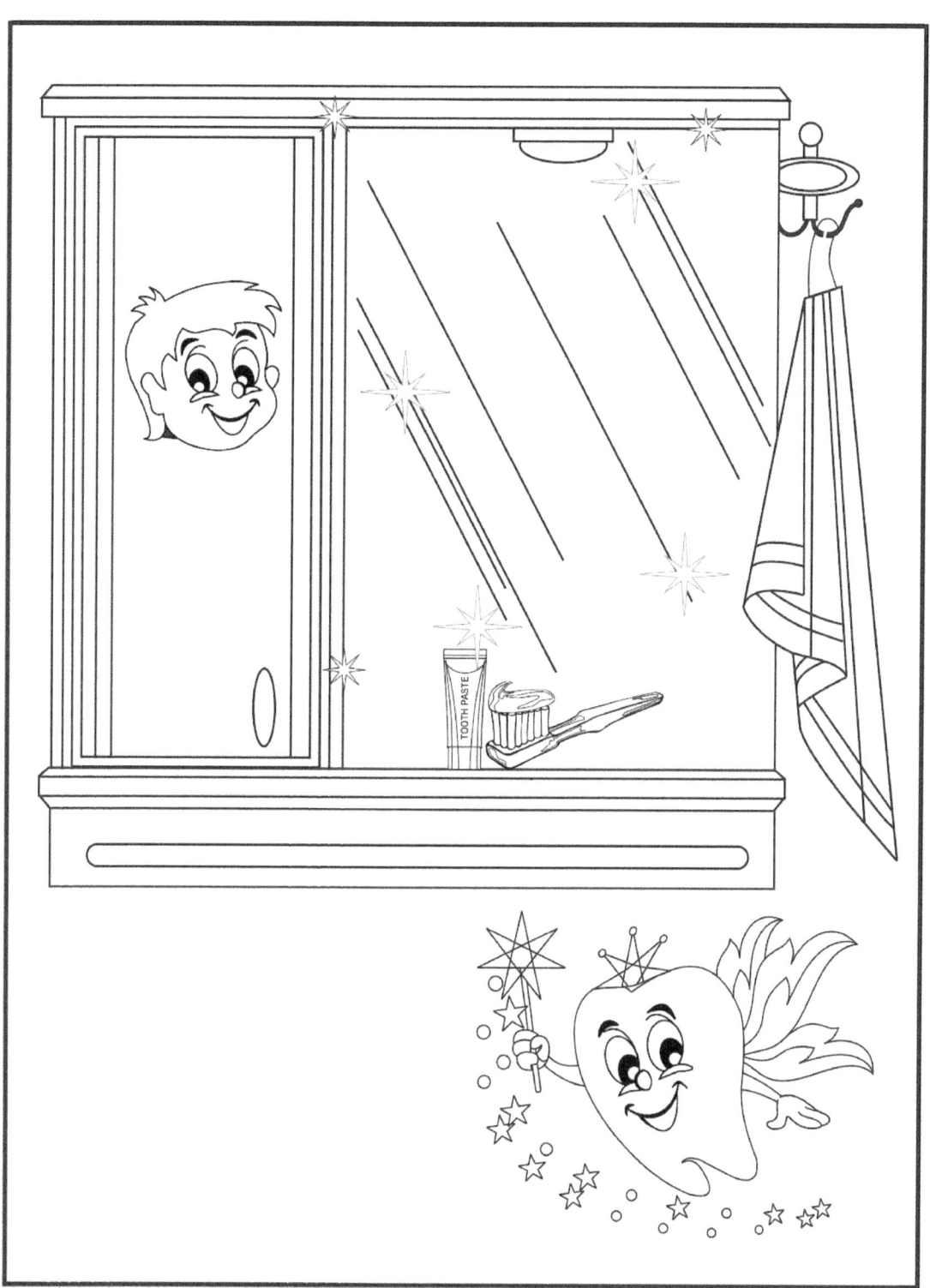

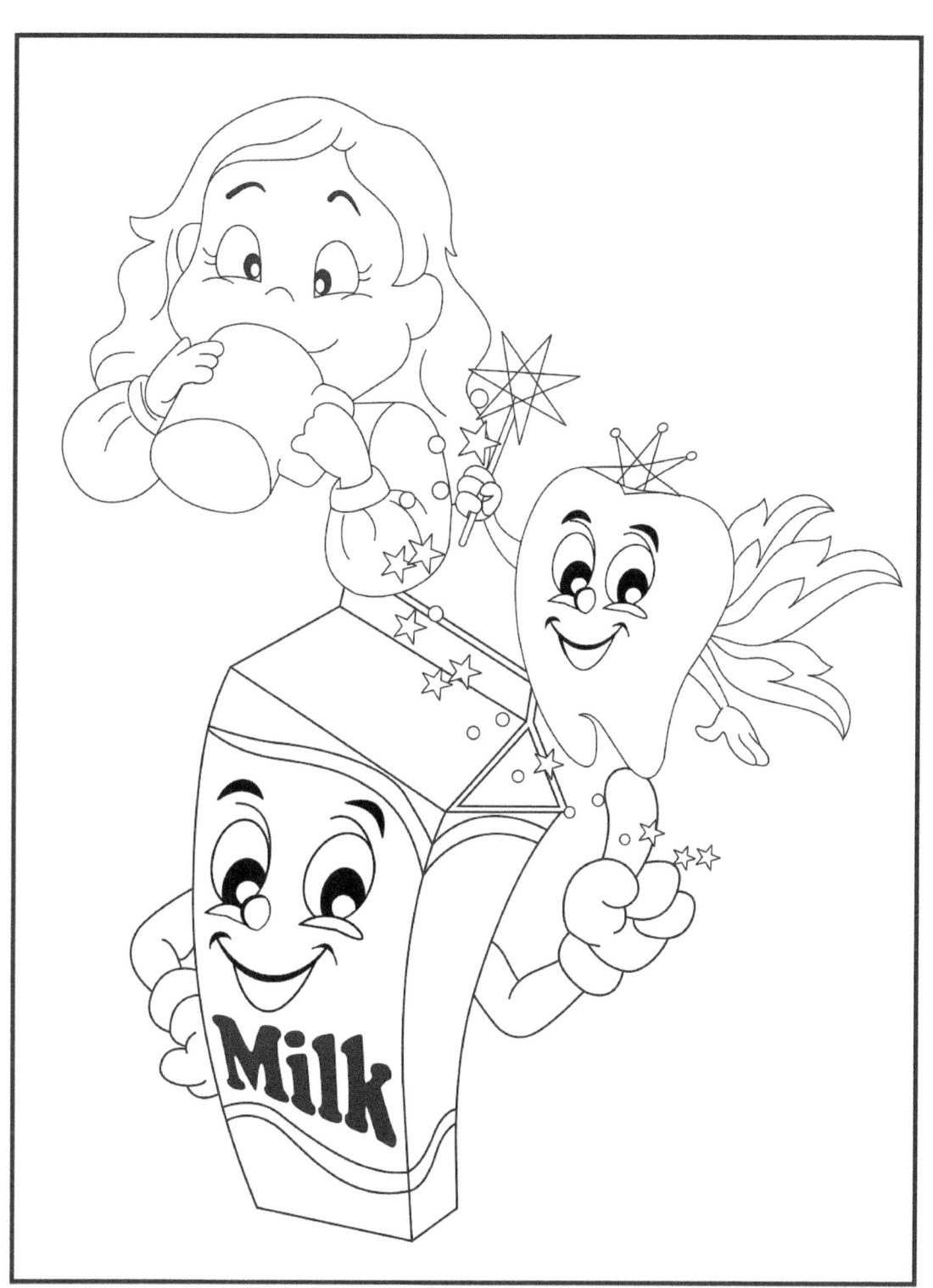

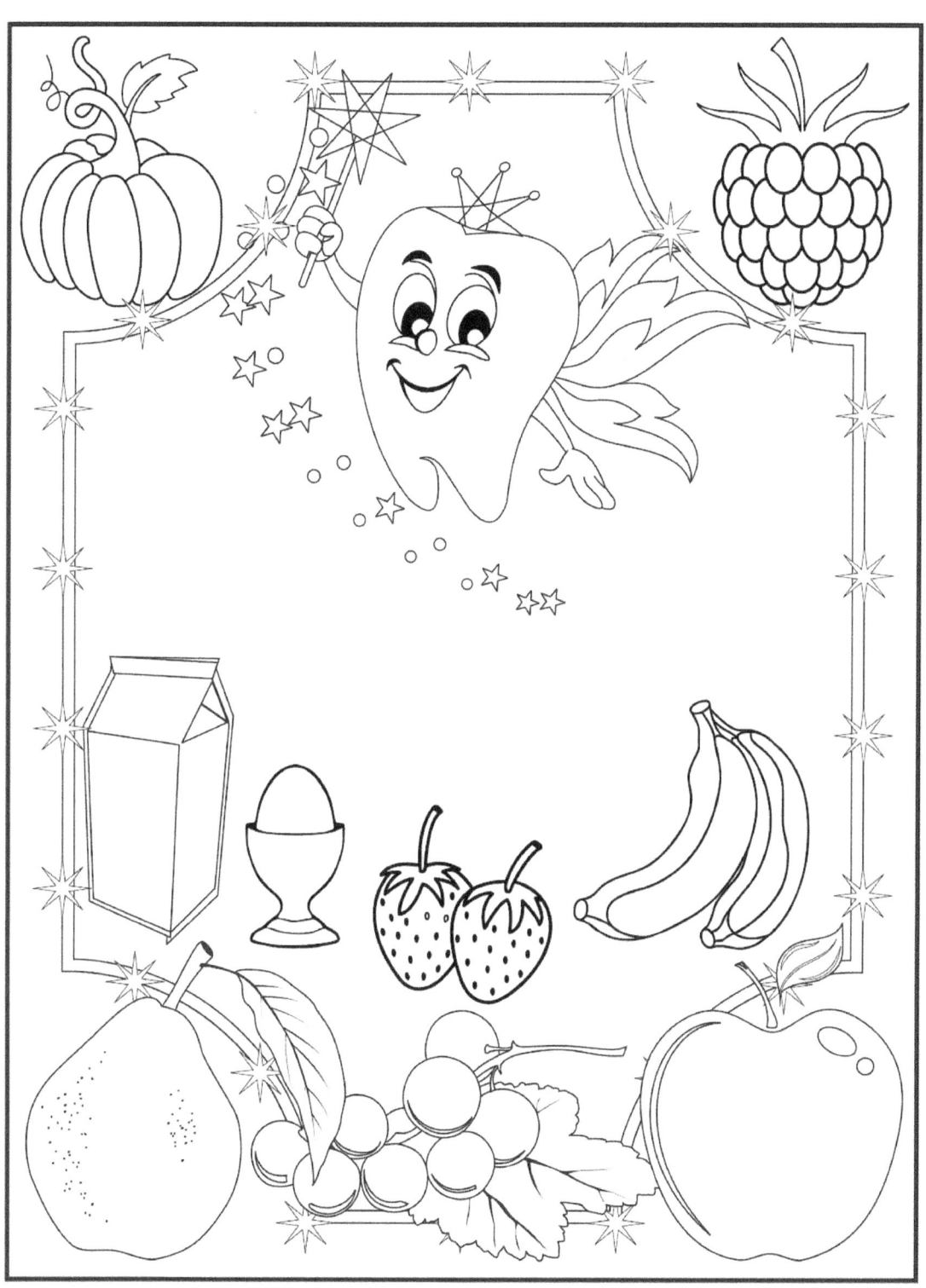

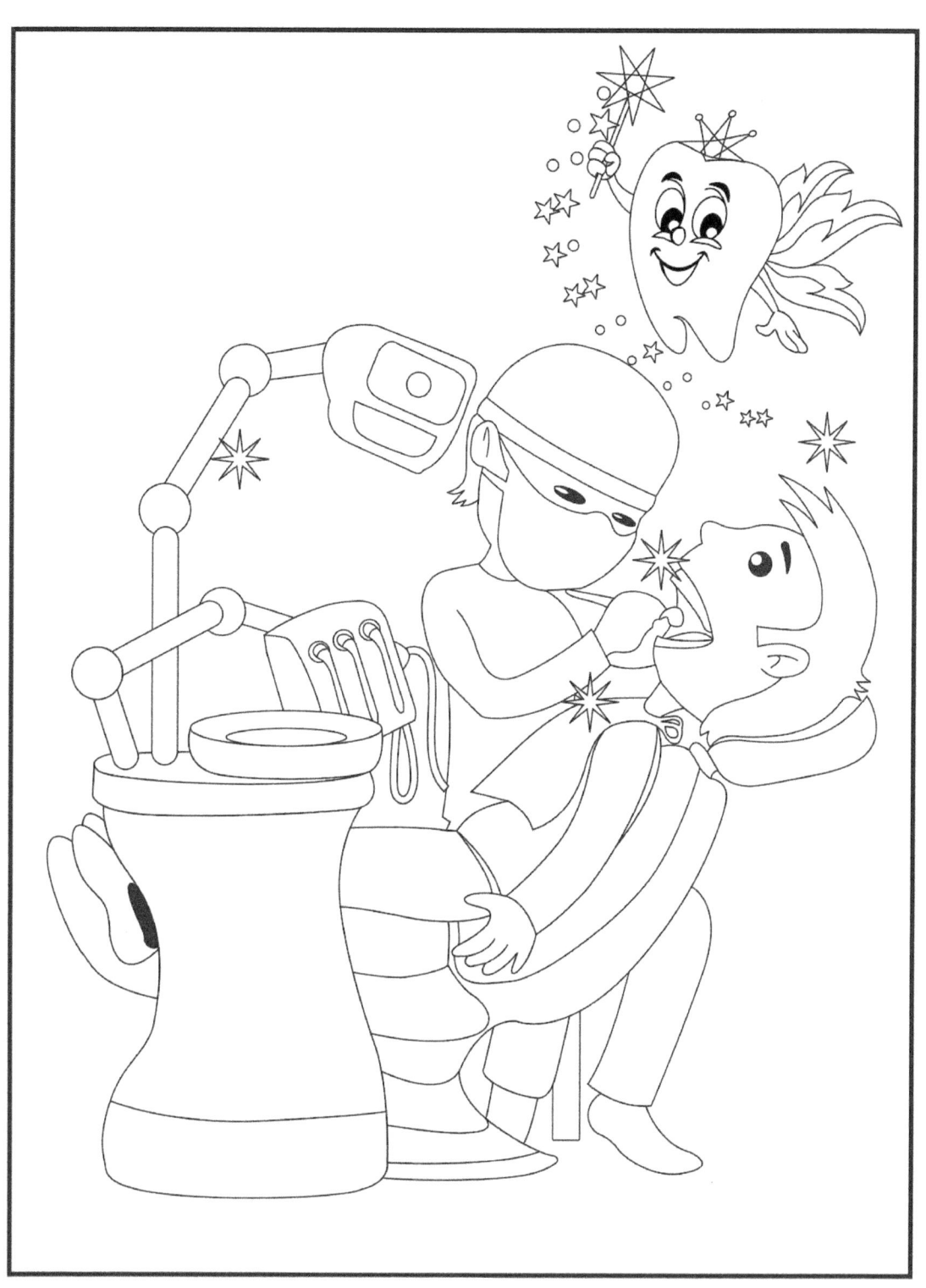

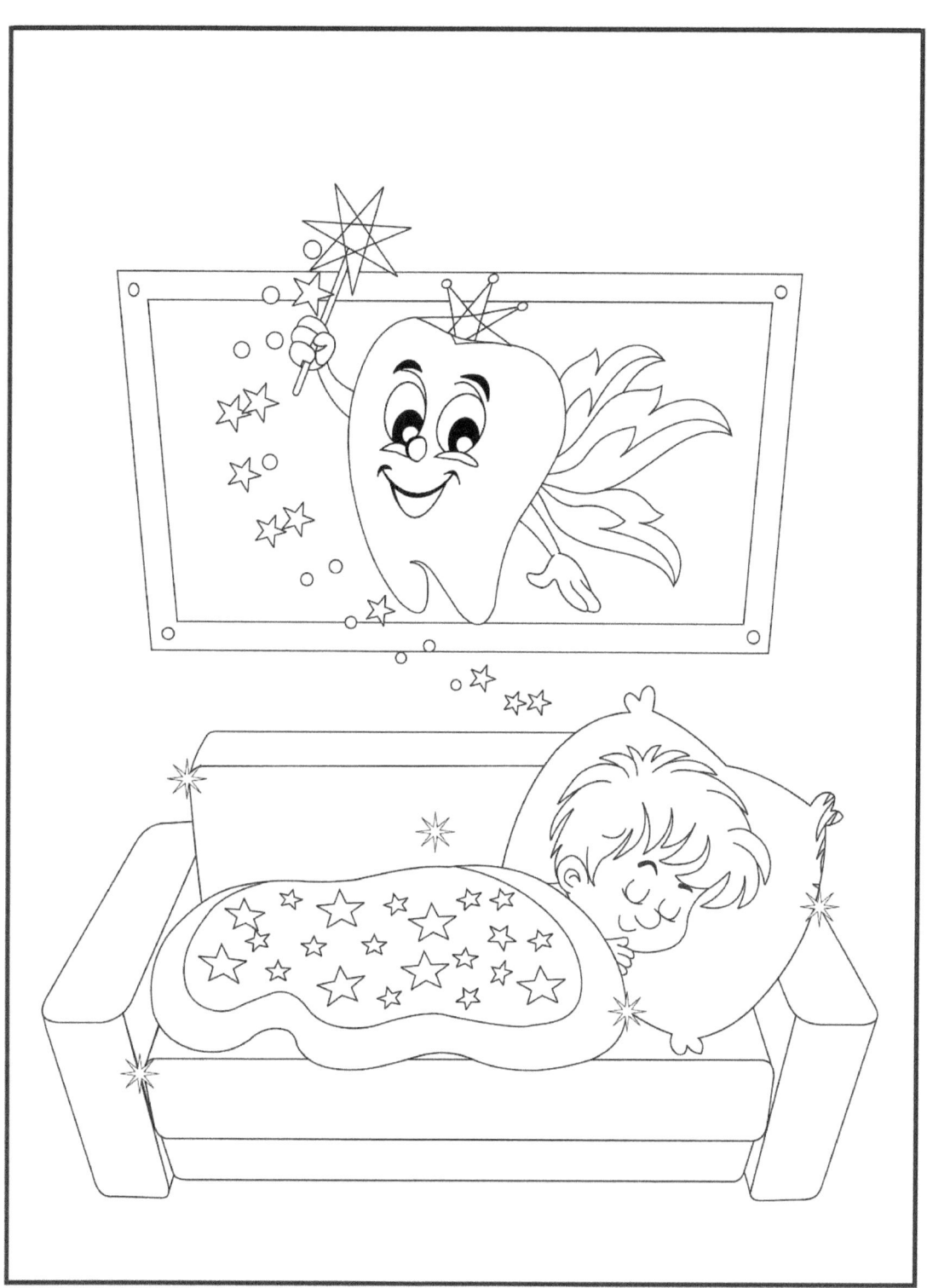

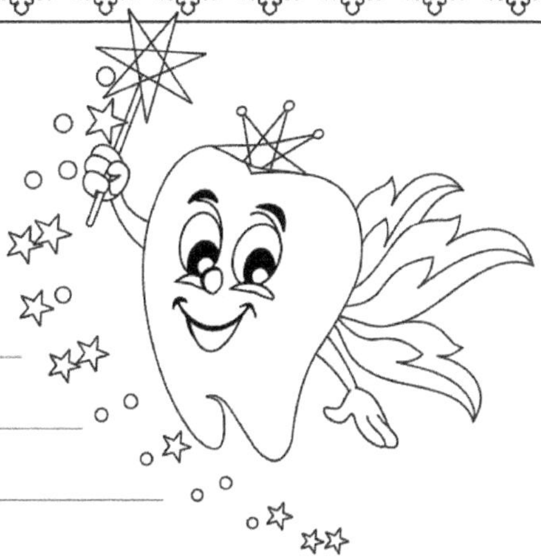

**Dear Tooth Fairy,**

_____

_____

_____

_____

_____

_____

_____

_____

_____

_____

_____

_____

_____

_____

_____

**From,**

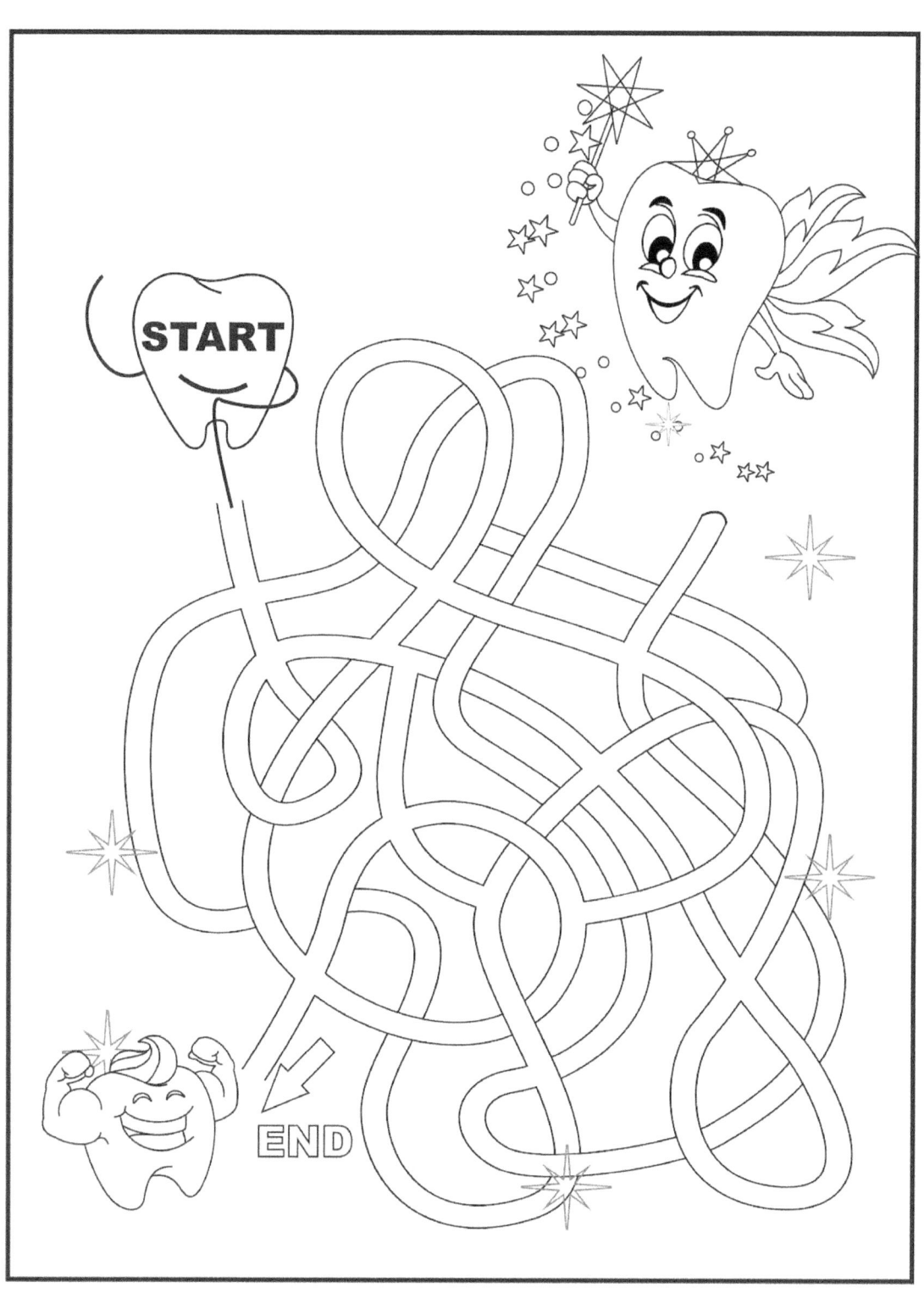

# Dental Word Search

```
K  J  A  R  V  F  P  D  D  L  Q  Y  T  Q  V        DENTIST
V  U  K  V  S  D  C  E  I  Z  R  L  V  C  R        TEETH
O  A  R  Z  I  Y  N  Y  S  O  I  W  H  S  F        TOOTH
U  V  T  O  O  T  H  H  K  B  B  A  E  L  Z        OKLAHOMA
M  K  K  D  I  N  Q  L  I  R  Y  N  A  B  A        GROVE
C  G  K  S  P  L  A  J  H  U  T  S  L  A  R        BRUSH
L  G  T  R  V  H  R  J  A  S  L  R  T  N  U        HEALTH
N  G  A  B  O  U  Q  P  U  H  S  T  H  W  S        FRUIT
Y  R  G  M  C  V  K  B  V  Z  V  A  U  H  P
X  O  A  J  N  B  U  Y  Q  V  F  K  L  I  S
M  V  H  X  P  W  F  D  T  J  K  N  K  C  R
K  E  S  X  D  R  E  V  M  E  T  Y  V  B  M
U  H  B  W  U  A  V  G  G  S  E  S  I  N  Y
W  I  R  I  P  H  H  Y  P  G  H  T  S  U  Q
P  W  T  V  Y  J  L  P  V  N  O  L  H  Q  J
```

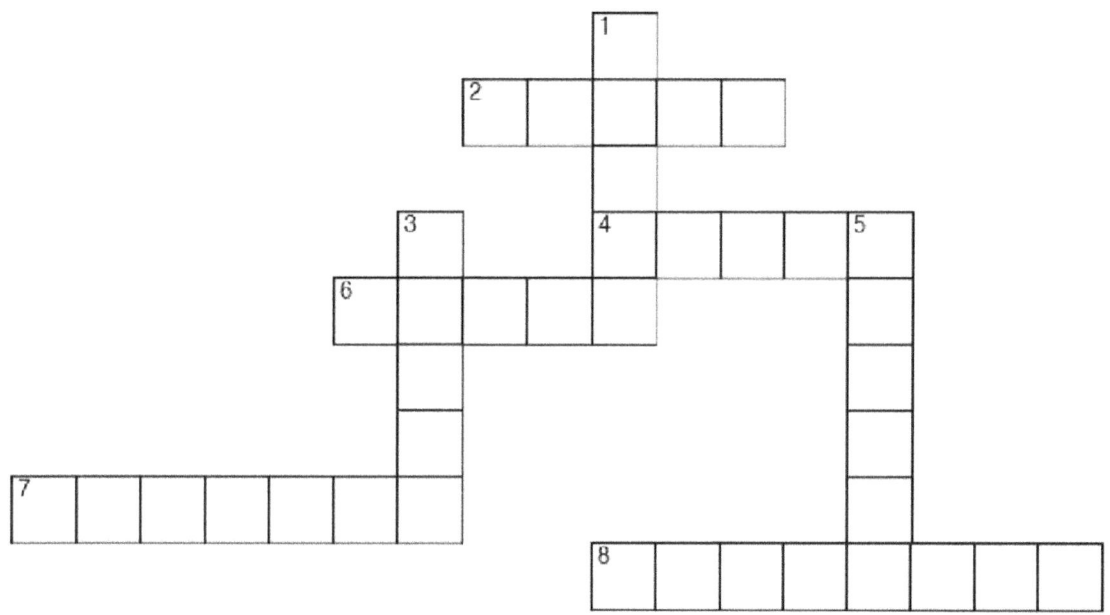

ACROSS
2 grove
4 teeth
6 brush
7 dentist
8 oklahoma

DOWN
1 tooth
3 fruit
5 health

# Thank you for trying the

# Karl Jobst Activity Book!

**Here's more about the man behind the book**

Karl Jobst, DDS, is a dentist who chose to build his start-of-the-art practice in Grove, Oklahoma. Grand Lake Dental is located quite close to Dr. Jobst's childhood home and is founded on the principle that providing patients with the highest level of dental care is of paramount importance. Dr. Jobst's commitment to continuing education, along with the staff he has assembled at Grand Lake Dental, is representative of the practice's foundational principle. As a result, patients have indeed come to expect access to the latest in dental technology as provided by a caring and committed team of dental professionals.

Founded in 1998, Grand Lake Dental quickly developed a reputation for always being on the cutting edge of technology. Even after graduating from the University of Tennessee College of Dental Medicine, Dr. Jobst continued to pursue opportunities to expand his skillset by completing postgraduate programs through the University of Southern California and the Las Vegas Institute. The efforts of Karl Jobst, DDS, in this regard have enabled him to offer innovative treatments representing a minimally invasive alternative to the traditional treatment options some patients perceive as causing discomfort.

A highly regarded dentist and the founder of an exceptionally successful dental practice, Dr. Jobst has enjoyed a professional career that has enabled him to help a great deal of people throughout the Grand Lake area. Through his volunteer efforts and his active membership in the church, Dr. Jobst has also endeavored to contribute a great deal more to the community beyond the exceptional dental services he provides at his practice.